Mediterranean Diet

7 Day Proven Step by Step Strategic Guide to a Healthier Stronger Heart and a Slimmer Sexier Waist for Life

Introduction

I want to thank you and congratulate you for downloading the book, *"Mediterranean Diet: Your 7 Day Proven Step by Step Strategic Guide to a Healthier Stronger Heart and a Slimmer Sexier Waist for Life"*.

This book contains proven steps and strategies on how to achieve a healthier life and a slimmer body by following the Mediterranean diet. This diet is not what you think it is. It isn't about a luxurious, upscale, fancy meal. It also isn't a 3-hour long feast with overflowing wine. The true Mediterranean diet is all about fresh food prepared in the simplest ways. And this diet can give you a lot of health benefits, including weight loss and a healthy heart.

To learn more about this diet and how it can help you, read this book today. You will also learn how to make the transition easier and less of a hassle. Read this book and get ready to transform your life.

Thanks again for downloading this book, I hope you enjoy it!

Table of Contents
Mediterranean Diet

Introduction

Chapter 1 Benefits of the Mediterranean Diet

Chapter 2 How to Start the Mediterranean Diet To Start Losing Weight

Chapter 3 The 7-Day Mediterranean Diet Plan

Chapter 4 General Food Guidelines for Health and Weight Loss

Chapter 5 Overview of the Mediterranean Diet

Conclusion

Chapter 1 Benefits of the Mediterranean Diet

There is a renewed attention and enthusiasm about the Mediterranean diet in recent years. A lot of researches found out that the diet is rich in nuts, fresh vegetables and fruits, olive oil and fish, providing protection against serious illnesses. Aside from that, it also helps in maintaining a healthy weight.

More specific health benefits include:

Protection from Type 2 Diabetes

Traditional Mediterranean diet is rich in fiber. The fiber slows down the rate of digestion of carbohydrates. This way, the blood sugar levels do not quickly shoot up and just as rapidly drop. Type 2 diabetes develops from rapid sugar-insulin spikes that occur frequently.

Protects against stroke and heart diseases

Modern, average meals are high in processed food and red meat. All these contribute to increasing one's risk in developing stroke and cardiovascular diseases. All these food are highly discouraged in the Mediterranean diet. Also, red wine is more preferred than drinking hard liquor. Research studies showed that red wine contains beneficial compounds that provide protective effects on the heart and the cardiovascular system.

Reduced risk of developing Parkinson's disease

The diet provides a substantial amount of antioxidants obtained from the abundance of fresh fruits and vegetables. These antioxidants provide a protective effect on the cells against damage from oxidative stress. Parkinson's disease develops from the degeneration or destruction of the nerve cells. By taking more antioxidants, the cells will have better protection against destruction. This also helps reduce the risk of Parkinson's by as much as 50%.

Reduced risk of developing Alzheimer's disease

Research found that following a Mediterranean diet improves the body's lipid profile. It improves the levels of cholesterol in the blood and promotes better ration between LDL and HDL. Also, blood sugar levels are better regulated. All these improvements are believed by experts to help in reducing a person's risk for developing Alzheimer's disease.

Reduced risk for cancers

Healthier eating practices help in preventing several types of cancer. Increased fiber intake helps reduce colon cancers. Antioxidants from fresh fruits and vegetables help in strengthening the cells against damage and cancer formation.

Vitamins and minerals help the body's organs to repair itself and recover faster and better, to prevent any cancer cells from developing within the damaged structures.

Improved musculoskeletal health

The diet is rich in natural vitamins, minerals and other essential nutrients that help keep the joints, muscle and the rest of the musculoskeletal system working well and free of pain. A study found that the nutrients supplied by the Mediterranean diet helps in reducing the elderly's risk for muscle weakness and frailty symptoms related to advancement of age.

Longer life

Because of the reduced risk for diseases such as cancer and heart attack, a person has a 20% reduction in death risk. That is, those who follow the Mediterranean diet enjoy longer, healthier lives.

Weight loss

All these healthy eating practices help lose excess weight and maintain it within the healthy range. Numerous researches on obesity found that frequent sugar and insulin spikes promote fat accumulation in the body and slow down metabolism and fat burning. Unhealthy trans fats and saturated fats from the average diet are not utilized by the body and are stored as added fats. Also, the chemicals from food processing such as the preservatives, flavor enhancers and stabilizers all contribute to an imbalance in the body that promotes obesity. Take all these out and the body is able to return to its normal and efficient metabolism and fat control. The net result is losing excess weight.

Chapter 2 - How to Start the Mediterranean Diet to Start Losing Weight

The Mediterranean diet is very different from what most people are used to eating. An average person's regular meal would be mostly meat, with lots of processed ingredients and cooked in butter or other unhealthy oils. Pasta comes from white carbohydrates and eaten in large servings. Vegetables and fruits are limited to a few slices that act more as garnish rather than a real part of the meal. All these have to be changed when choosing to follow the Mediterranean diet for health.

To keep from getting overwhelmed and avoid feeling deprived, start by making small substitutions. The transition is easier this way. Remember, the Mediterranean diet is not a one-time only kind of die. It is more of a lifestyle. Prepare to follow this diet for a lifetime, and not just on a short-term basis.

•   When ordering pizza or pasta, choose the flavors that have more vegetables than meats. For example, order pizza with more olives and mushrooms rather than the all-meat pepperoni pizza. When ordering pasta, choose tomato-based or oil-based (olive oil) sauces rather than the cream-based ones. Skip the meatballs.

•   Substitute red meats with fish or poultry. Set aside at least 2 fish nights each week and gradually increase in frequency.

•   Set aside a meatless day each week and go for a vegetarian meal.

•   Substitute all other fats with olive oil. Sautéing vegetables? Omit the butter and use olive oil instead. Brush grilled or baked foods with olive oil instead of butter or margarine.

•   Choose low-fat versions of dairy products such as yogurt and low fat-cheese.

•   Have fresh fruits for dessert. Use whatever fruit is in season.

•   When in doubt, choose foods that were prepared in the simplest ways.

•   Choose whole grain breads and pastas instead of those made with refined flour (white flour).

More specific substitutions that can help make the transition smoother include the following examples:

- Quinoa instead of white rice

- Whole wheat tortillas instead of white bread

- Stir-fried vegetables (in olive oil) instead of stir-fried meat

- Vegetables slices (cucumbers, carrots, celery or broccoli) for snacks instead of chips and crackers

- Bean dip instead of ranch dip

- Yogurt instead of ice cream

- Glass of red wine instead of beer

Chapter 3 - The 7-Day Mediterranean Diet Plan

For full commitment on the Mediterranean diet and to get the most benefits, here is a 7-day Menu plan. This diet plan can help in getting started on achieving weight loss with a side of better health.

Day 1

Breakfast: Pancakes made with whole wheat or buckwheat flour (instead of white flour) and fat-free milk and yogurt instead of regular whole milk. Serve with a cup of fresh fruits such as blueberries or strawberries.

Lunch: Chickpea Salad using fresh chickpeas, with diced onions, green peppers, black olives and romaine lettuce leaves. Drizzle with olive oil or make vinaigrette by adding vinegar (white or apple cider vinegar)

Dinner: Grilled chicken marinated in fat-free Italian dressing

Snack: Wholewheat or crispbread crackers with hummus dip

Day 2

Breakfast: Granola and Yogurt Parfait with fresh raspberries. Just layer everything in a wide-mouth glass, starting with granola and ending with the fresh fruits.

Lunch: Grilled tomato with mozzarella Sandwich

Dinner: Vegetable Pot Pie, use whole wheat or other whole grain flour for the crust

Snack: Fresh berries salad. Mix different berries such as raspberries, blueberries and blackberries. Drizzle with ½ tablespoon honey or add to low-fat yogurt.

Day 3

Breakfast: Vegetable Omelet

Lunch: Fresh Basil, tomato and feta cheese sandwich

Dinner: Grilled sea bass, drizzled with olive oil and served over a bed of baby arugula leaves.

Snack: Cucumber and carrot sticks with chickpea dip

Day 4

Breakfast: Low-fat granola with fresh banana slices

Lunch: Grilled chicken breast with olive oil served with steamed baby carrots and artichokes

Dinner: Vegetable frittata with blanched spinach leaves drizzled with balsamic vinegar

Snack: Cucumber slices and carrot sticks with sour cream dip

Day 5

Breakfast: low fat yogurt with whole grain cereals

Lunch: Pita sandwich made with fresh vegetable slices (cucumbers, tomatoes and carrots) and baked turkey breast. Dressing is garlic yogurt. Just mix minced garlic to low fat yogurt. Add ground black pepper if desired.

Dinner: Baked chicken with baby potatoes and baby carrots with a side of steamed artichokes and arugula leaves

Snack: Use garlic yogurt dressing as dip for graham crackers

Day 6

Breakfast: Whole wheat bagel with natural peanut butter spread

Lunch: Whole wheat thin crust pizza with toppings of mushrooms, olives, capers, fresh onions and bell peppers

Dinner: lamb souvlaki with couscous

Snack: Fresh fruit smoothie topped with a handful of toasted pine nuts

Day 7

Breakfast: Pita bread with ricotta cheese spread

Lunch: Shrimp salad with fresh tomatoes, basil leaves and salad greens

Dinner: Pan-grilled salmon n olive oil, with balsamic vinegar dressing served with couscous and fresh salad greens drizzled with olive oil

Snack: a handful of toasted nuts such as pistachio or toasted sunflower seeds

Notice that there are more fresh fruits and vegetables, fish and grains. There are limited meats and processed foods, as well as dairy products. The Mediterranean diet incorporates key elements that put more focus on making healthier food choices and adopting a better approach to food and eating. These elements help in various capacities to promote heart health and weight loss.

Chapter 4 - General Food Guidelines for Health and Weight Loss

Over the years, the traditional Mediterranean diet was modified so much that it no longer resembled the healthy eating practice it once were. In 1993, a team consisting of an organization called Oldways, the European Office of the World Health Organization (WHO), and Harvard School of Public Health, introduced the Mediterranean Diet Pyramid. This was a graphic representation of what the classic Mediterranean is.

This pyramid was formulated by studying what a real, traditional Mediterranean meal consists of. Modern nutrition research conducted by top notch universities and top rated researchers in the field provided scientific backing of what the pyramid includes.

Dietary traditions observed in the island of Crete, as well as those in Greece and the southern portion of Italy, during the 1960s were used as a major basis for the development of the Mediterranean diet pyramid. This was the time when these places suffered poverty, which made people turn to growing their own food. These regions had very limited access to modern-day food such as processed foods. All they had to eat most of the time were garden produced and those caught from the sea. This period also saw the highest adult life expectancy in the region compared to the rest of the world. People enjoyed better health, with the least rates on cardiovascular diseases, despite limited access to medical services.

Studies found that the widely considered "poor diet" was actually better for health. The region in those times did not enjoy the convenience of modernized food, such as processed meats and processed foods, instant meals and other artificially preserved and manufactured foods. They ate fresh produce such as fruits and vegetables, beans, nuts and grains. They also used olive oils that they themselves produced in the traditional manner, not from manufacturing plants. They are more fish caught fresh from the sea, since the area is near the Mediterranean Sea. They had limited dairy product intake as well as meats from cows and pigs because the area was not very well suited for raising livestock.

MEDITERRANEAN DIET PYRAMID

This pyramid is now the standard to healthy diets in order to obtain optimum health through making the right food choices and eating the right amounts. Years of study and research have solidified the effectiveness of this diet pyramid, which is now widely accepted as the "Gold Standard when it comes to eating for lifelong optimum health.

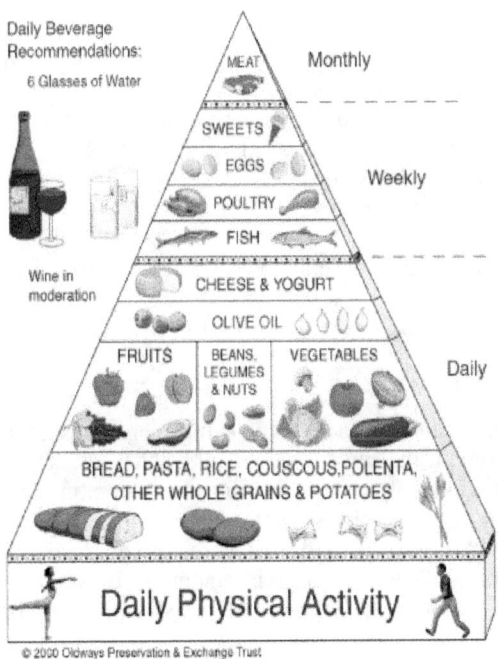

The Traditional Healthy
Mediterranean Diet Pyramid

Daily Beverage Recommendations:

6 Glasses of Water

Wine in moderation

Monthly

MEAT

SWEETS

EGGS

POULTRY

Weekly

FISH

CHEESE & YOGURT

OLIVE OIL

FRUITS | BEANS, LEGUMES & NUTS | VEGETABLES

Daily

BREAD, PASTA, RICE, COUSCOUS, POLENTA, OTHER WHOLE GRAINS & POTATOES

Daily Physical Activity

As seen in the pyramid, the lower half includes those that should be done or eaten on a daily basis. The upper half of the pyramid is further divided into 2. The lower category includes things that can be eaten on a weekly basis, in moderate amounts and only for a few days. The topmost category includes what should be eaten on a monthly basis, a few times only and in moderation. This pyramid also summarizes the key elements or focus of the entire diet:

Focus: Physical Activity

Daily physical activity is at the base. This means that it should be given the same importance as what is given on food. Weight loss not only involves eating the right foods. It also involves burning excess stored fat. Physical activity also helps in better regulation of fat metabolism, as well as better fat use.

Physical activity on a regular basis is done at levels that promote wellbeing and healthy weight. This means appropriate physical activity for each individual health status.

Focus: Carbohydrates

Next at the bottom of the diet pyramid is eating carbohydrates from healthier sources. Carbohydrates constitute a huge percentage of daily food intake. It should be from whole grains such as whole grain pasta and bread, polenta, couscous, and rice. Potatoes are also good sources of carbohydrates. These provide quick energy but do not cause sugar and insulin spikes that promote weight gain and health problems like diabetes. Next level of the diet pyramid includes vegetables, nuts, legumes, beans and fruits. These are main sources of minerals, vitamins and antioxidants that help in regulating metabolism s well as promote better cellular health and function. Olive oil is the main fat source, practically used in preparing all the rest of the foods in the Mediterranean diet pyramid. Cheese and dairy are taken in moderation each day.

Focus: Food from Plants

The primary focus of the Mediterranean diet is on eating more foods from plants. This includes vegetables and fruits, nuts, seeds, legumes and whole grains. These are rich in fiber that helps in regulating sugar and insulin, preventing spikes that promote weight gain and health problems. These plant-based foods are also rich in fiber that help in controlling hunger and cravings, as well as promote fullness and satisfaction from meals. Fiber also helps in binding excess and bad lipids from the blood and brings it out of the body via the digestive system. Fibers also act as mops that attract toxins and bring them out for excretion. Removal of toxins helps in improving metabolism, which can help in faster weight loss.

On the average, people who followed the traditional diet get 6 or more servings per day of vegetables and fruits that are rich in anti-oxidants. For best benefits, these are eaten fresh and whole, or at least, minimally processed. These are taken as part of meals or as snacks. There are a variety of vegetable and fruit salads that can be eaten for meals, desserts and snacks. Fresh fruits are served daily as the typical dessert. Sweets that contain sugar (or honey) and saturated fats are limited to only a few times each week.

Grains included in the Mediterranean diet are whole grains. These are often made into bead, but without the unhealthy trans fats. Breads from whole grains are important in this diet. These, however, are eaten as they are, without any fillings or spreads. Or, the bread is simply dipped in olive oil, not smeared with margarine or butter that is rich in trans fats or saturated fats. Also, whole grains are eaten in the form of whole grain rice, cereals and pastas.

Nuts are often taken for granted in other kinds of diet. In the Mediterranean diet, nuts are considered sources of healthy fats. These are also high in proteins and fibers that provide lots of health benefits. They make good crunchy texture for meals. These also make great, handy, hassle-free snacks. However, they are also high in calories so nuts should be taken in moderation. Eat no more than a handful each day. Also, avoid nuts that have been heavily salted, candied or roasted in honey. Nuts can be taken as nut butters. Although, choose the naturally made one, such as natural peanut butter, and not the butters that contain unhealthy hydrogenated fats. Tahini is a healthy nut-based dip or spread for breads. Tahini is blended sesame seeds.

Focus: Healthy Fats

Not all fats are bad for health. There are few that can actually be good for the body. In fact, the diet does not put a limit on total daily fat consumption. What the diet highly advises against is the use of hydrogenated oils (or trans fats) and saturated fats. These 2 kinds of fats are very unhealthy and known to be closely linked to the development of heart diseases.

Mediterranean diet is known for its extensive use of olive oil. Lots of research found the same results- olive oil is healthy. It contains healthy monounsaturated fatty acids that provide protective benefits on the heart and the blood vessels. Monounsaturated fats help keep the body healthy by reducing the levels of LDL (low density lipoprotein). Using extra virgin olive oils (EVOO) adds more benefits. This oil has the least processing done, which means that it has more of the natural plant compounds intact. These plant compounds have potent antioxidant effects that add to the oil's health benefits.

Other healthy oils used in the diet include oils from certain nuts and canola oil. These oils are rich in linolenic acid, which is a type of healthy omega-3 fatty acids. These also contain a good amount of unsaturated fats that are also healthy for the body. In the body, omega-3 fats help in lowering triglyceride levels and reducing blood clotting. These are linked to decreased risk for heart attacks, better regulation of blood pressure and improved health status of the blood vessels. Other sources of healthy fats and omega-3 fats include cold water fishes like mackerel, albacore tuna, sardines, herring, salmon and lake trout. Incidentally, Mediterranean meals incorporate large amounts of olive oil and lots of fish.

Focus: Dairy and Processed Foods

Dairy is also consumed in limited amounts. Choose the healthier, low-fat versions such as low-fat cheese, skim milk and fat-free yogurt. Minimize consumption of high fat products such as ice cream, cheese and whole or 2% milk.

Focus: Fish

Fish is another healthy source of protein. The Mediterranean diet includes more fish than red meat and poultry. The diet recommends eating fish for a minimum of 2 times per week. Healthy fish choices include tuna, mackerel, salmon, herring and trout. How these are cooked is also important. Avoid breaded fried fish. It's better to broil, bake or grill it. These are more convenient methods of cooking fish, as well healthier.

Focus: Limit Red Meat,

First off, these are the expensive stuff. Traditional Mediterranean diet is supposedly the diet of the poor people, who couldn't afford the expensive red meat, processed food and dairy. So they had to stick to whatever food they produce from their own gardens and from what they can catch from the sea. The diet may be considered as "poor folks' diet" but it was proven over and over as the healthy way to go. So, limit the red meat. Choose the lean portions, in small serving sizes (about the same size as that of a deck of cards). Red meat consumption is limited to a few times each month, not on a regular, daily basis. Recent research recommends limiting red meat consumption to not more than 12-16 ounces or 340-450grams each month. Lean cuts of red meat are more preferable.

Better yet, substitute red meat with fish and poultry. Avoid meats that have been processed and contain high amounts of fats such as bacon and sausages.

Focus: Wine

One of the attractive elements (for some, that is) of the Mediterranean diet is the incorporation of alcohol. What other healthy diet gives a nod on drinking wine? For years, there are several studies done that tried to determine whether alcohol is good or bad for the body. Most studies show that alcohol in moderation reduces the risk for the development of heart diseases.

The Mediterranean diet includes regular consumption of wine, specifically red wine. The intake is moderate, though. Wine consumption is limited to a daily maximum of 5 ounces or 148 milliliters of wine for women regardless of age and for men who are older than 65 years old. For younger men, daily maximum is at 10ounces or 296 milliliters. Consuming more than this recommendation is increasing one's risk for a few types of cancer and other health problems.

It isn't, however, a must to drink wine when following the Mediterranean diet. People who do not take alcohol before the diet need not have to drink. Also, people who have history of alcoholism or a tendency to become one are highly discouraged to incorporate alcohol in the diet. Remember, red wine can help but is not absolutely necessary when following the diet.

The above components of the Mediterranean diet pyramid are based on the classic diet in the original region (i.e., southern Italy, Crete and Greece). Research on this diet continues and the current results are used in modifying any applicable areas of the pyramid to better cater to the changing trends in health and nutrition.

Updated Mediterranean Diet Pyramid

In November 2008, The Mediterranean Diet Conference celebrated its 15th anniversary. During the conference, a few major updates were incorporated by the Scientific Advisory Board into the classic diet pyramid. The changes were focused on placing all the plant foods under one group in order to give it a higher visual importance on the pyramid. The change was aimed at drawing more attention to the vital role that plant foods play in the Mediterranean diet.

Another change made to the pyramid was the addition of spices and herbs. The main reason for the inclusion was for taste and health. Herbs and spices improve the taste of food. These also contain healthy and beneficial compounds that can boost the health benefits of the Mediterranean diet. Aside from this, the herbs and spices play a role in giving national identities to the different Mediterranean cuisines.

Also, the scientific committee adjusted the placement of shellfish and fish on the diet pyramid. Research found that these foods have positive benefits when eaten at least twice each week because of its rich content of omega-3 fatty acids. This healthy fat has a protective effect on the cardiovascular system, as well as helps improve the body's lipid profile.

Chapter 5 - Overview of the Mediterranean Diet

The Mediterranean diet is an ancient diet that has proven to be as effective and relevant in today's world. Mediterranean diet quickly evokes an Italian meal of pasta and pizza or a Greek meal of pita and hummus. Most people associate this diet to a 3-hour meal of lasagna, gyros, racks of lamb, pizza, huge loaves of white bread and falafel. Then, everything is washed down with overflowing wine. But, the real Mediterranean diet is a meal consisting heavily of vegetables and fruits, with olive oil, seafood and hearty grains. It is based in the traditional diet of Greece, southern Italy and Crete during the 1960s.

This is based on a study found that people living in these areas had "deprived" meals but enjoyed higher rates of cardiovascular health, with the lowest rates of chronic diseases compared to the rest of the world at that time. Older studies, especially one made after World War by a team from the Mayo Clinic found that men in Crete who fared on "poorer, meager" meals of vegetables and fishes had much better cardiovascular health compared to men living in richer countries who were considered well fed. The research team correlated the diet of fresh vegetables and fruits with healthier seafood provided better protection against cardiovascular problems.

Aside from the homegrown and fresh food, the health benefits of the Mediterranean diet are also related to the entire approach to eating and healthy living. Daily exercise (i.e., farming, fishing, walking), deep appreciation and right approach to food and eating, as well as eating meals with others all work together to achieve a healthy body.

MYTH BUSTING ABOUT THE MEDITERRANEAN DIET

Aside from the misconception on what actually constitute a Mediterranean diet, there are a few other myths regarding the diet. These need to be addressed in order to get the full benefits of following the diet:

Myth #1: Mediterranean diet is expensive

Remember that the Mediterranean diet is the diet of poor farming and fisherfolk in the Mediterranean region. Hence, it does not really make sense to think that this diet is an expensive one. Also, the main protein sources are less expensive. In the Mediterranean diet, the proteins come from legumes, beans and lentils, which cost much less than meats. The rest of the meal consists of fresh fruits, whole grains and other plants. These are less expensive compared to meals consisting of processed foods, cheese and meat.

Myth #2: More wine means getting more health benefits

People think that if drinking a glass of wine promotes good heart health, then drinking 3 means 3 times healthier. The thing with wine is that it has healthy benefits in moderate amounts. If taken in large amounts, negative effects occur. Moderate wine consumption means 1 drink a day for women and 2 drinks a day for men. These is amounts provide a protective effect on the heart and the rest of the cardiovascular system. More than these recommended amounts, the effects would be opposite. It will have a negative effect on cardiovascular health, as well as on the liver.

Myth #3: Large servings of pasta and bread is how to go Mediterranean

Over the years, the Mediterranean diet has been reinvented and no longer within its original context. Pasta is part of the meal but not in the large servings that they are today. Originally, pasta in the Mediterranean diet is only a side dish, served in small portions and not as a main course. It is just about a half- to 1-cup serving. The rest consists of small meat portions, vegetables, salads and, sometimes, a small slice of bread.

Myth #4: Traditional Mediterranean diet is a weight loss diet

While the diet greatly helps, this isn't the one shot deal. Eating healthy is helping the body metabolize food more efficiently. The right foods also provide the right nutrients for the body to keep it healthy. However, it takes more than just eating the right kind of foods to lose weight. It takes regular exercise. People in the Mediterranean area had to walk up and down the steep hills in their area several times a day. They also tend to their animals and gardens all day. Hence, they get daily exercise aside from the healthy eating practices.

Myth #5: Mediterranean diet is all about food

Food is definitely a huge part of the Mediterranean diet but that's not all of it. It is more of a lifestyle. People eat with friends and family, enjoying the food as well as the company. They do not eat in front of a TV or eat in hurry. They take their time in eating, helping them digest the food better.

Conclusion

Thank you again for downloading this book!

Putting it all together

The Mediterranean diet is a delicious and healthy way to eat. Many people who switch to this style of eating say they'll never eat any other way.

Research has shown that the traditional Mediterranean diet reduces the risk of heart disease. In fact, an analysis of more than 1.5 million healthy adults demonstrated that following a Mediterranean diet was associated with a reduced risk of death from heart disease and cancer, as well as a reduced incidence of Parkinson's and Alzheimer's diseases.

Finally, if you enjoyed this book, then I'd like to ask you for a favor, would you be kind enough to leave a review for this book on Amazon? It'd be greatly appreciated!

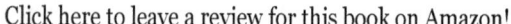

Click here to leave a review for this book on Amazon!

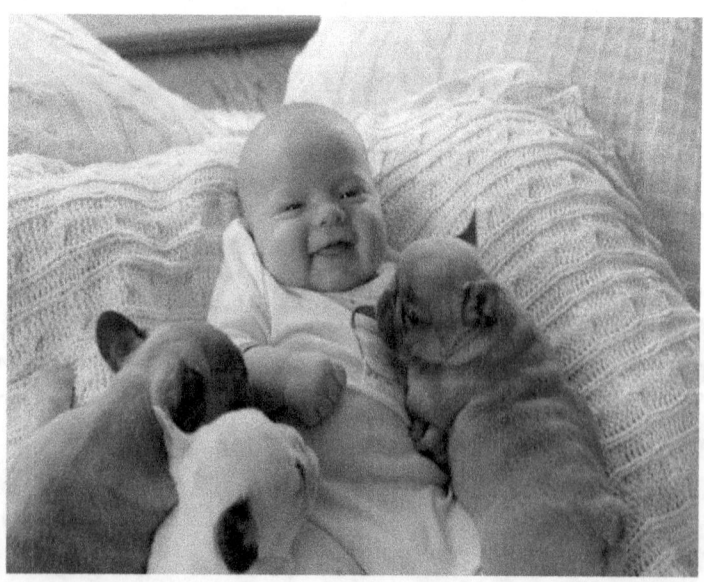

Thank you and good luck!

Check out my other Best Selling Books Below!!

Preview From Best Selling Author Jessica Virna "Hormone Reset Diet"

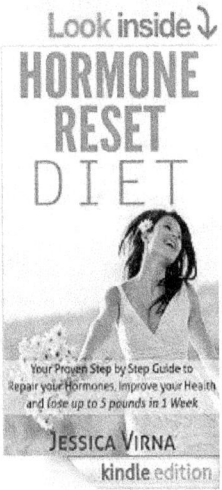

Chapter 1: Hormonal Imbalance: The Root Cause of Weight Loss Problems

Have you ever wondered why none of the dietary programs you have tried really worked well for you? Do you still gain weight despite all your hard work in keeping yourself fit? Do you easily feel stressed out with simple things? If you answered "yes" to all these questions, then you have failed to address the real root cause of the problem—hormonal imbalance.

Here are some questions that you need to ask yourself first to help determine if you have imbalanced hormones or not:

- Do you usually feel a strong urge to eat sweets or carbs at 3pm?
- Do you find it difficult to get yourself out of bed in the morning?
- Do you easily get irritated even by simple things?
- Do have mood swings?
- Do you experience pre-menstrual syndrome every month?
- Do you have trouble getting a good night's sleep?

- Is your skin dull and dry?
- Do you have a belly fat that you can't seem to get rid of no matter what you do?
- Do you always feel bloated after every meal?

If your answer is "yes" to all of these questions, then your hormone levels are not balanced. Fortunately, this book was written specifically for you.

Women are more susceptible to problems pertaining to hormones. No matter how little we eat or how healthy our diet is, if it doesn't balance out hormonal misfires then the efforts will be wasted for nothing. There are different signs of hormonal imbalances and often women fail to recognize that.

- Pre-menstrual syndrome
- Irritability and mood swings over little things
- Extra weight hanging around the waist/belly area
- Excessive cravings for sugar
- Easily stressed out
- Difficulty sleeping
- Overwhelming feeling

Women need to know that hormones control nearly all aspects of losing weight. They affect your appetite, food cravings, fat storage, food patterns and even gut bacteria. This means that when there's hormonal imbalance, nothing will work out well for you unless you address this problem first. Eliminating junk foods and exercising regularly have always been the experts' advice on losing weight, but with hormones getting all fired up, losing weight will be difficult.

Click Here to Check out the Rest of "The Hormone Reset Diet" on Amazon

Or go to: **http://amzn.to/1HhshKh**

Preview Of "Anti Inflammatory Diet"

Look inside ↓

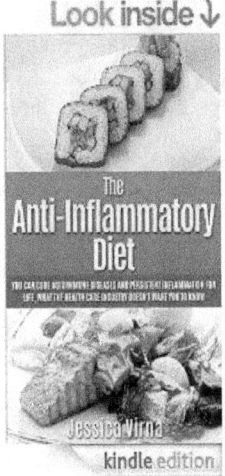

kindle edition

Chapter 1: What Is the Anti-Inflammatory Diet?

The Anti-Inflammatory Diet was originally invented by Dr. Weil, a nutritionist and diet expert. Often said to be almost similar to the Mediterranean Diet and the Zone Diet, but what makes it different is that it involves a lot of fish oil.

The Anti-Inflammatory Diet isn't just about protecting yourself from diseases—it's also about maintaining your ideal weight, too! When you're under this diet, you can expect that you'll easily be able to lose weight in a natural manner.

But what exactly is this about and what could Fish Oil, amongst others, do?

Benefits of Fish Oil
Fish Oil is a good source of Omega-3 Fatty Acids that could strengthen the overall condition of the mind, heart, and immune system in general. This is important because the human body cannot naturally produce Omega-3 Fatty Acids, and a lack of it would therefore bring forth a lot of deficiencies.

More so, one of the main reasons why you need Fish Oil and why the Anti-Inflammatory Diet is around is because it could protect you against Mitochondrial Dysfunction.

Mitochondrial Dysfunction
Mitochondrial Dysfunction results from a combination of erroneous stressors and aging that naturally bring forth a lot of diseases. When a person undergoes

this, his cell walls are damaged—which therefore means that he easily becomes susceptible to a lot of negative medical conditions.

Another thing that happens is that free radicals make their way to the body, which then weakens cell membranes, and could bring about heightened levels of Uric Acid that could cause hypertension, slow metabolic rate, and a lot of heart problems.

When these things happen, Chronic Inflammation could take over the body.

Chronic Inflammation

As mentioned earlier, chronic inflammation could be the basis of a lot of dangerous diseases that could ruin the body—mentally, physically, and emotionally. What makes it really scary is the fact that there aren't concrete medical tests that could really check for Chronic Inflammation. Sure, there are cancer tests, heart disease tests, and more, but no one could be able to tell whether you're easily susceptible to these problems or not—and that's why in this case, prevention really proves to be better than cure.

Before you get to know what you should and shouldn't eat, it would be good to first know about what may cause Chronic Inflammation. There are 3 main categories for this, and these are:

1. Physical. This can come from one or more of the following:

Blunt or Penetrating Skin Injuries. It often happens when the injured person picks off scabs from his body.

Burns and Frostbite. These are two extreme effects of the weather, or of accidents that may cause a lot of pain and swelling for the afflicted person.

Debris, dirt, and splinters. Oftentimes, people neglect the way they experience these things and may sometimes be too lazy to take away unnecessary particles from their bodies, and thus, it leads to other diseases and worsening skin conditions.

Ionizing Radiation. There are certain diseases that can be cured by radiation, such as Cancer, but then again, it also has really adverse side effects, such as causing chronic inflammation.

Trauma. When someone gets into a terrible accident, swelling may be induced more and so he may suffer from chronic inflammation.

2. Biological, which is often related to reaction formations in the brain, and could be caused by the following:

Hypersensitivity. Auto-immune Disorders, and other complex immune diseases are often experienced by those who have hypersensitive immune systems.

Pathogenic Infection. Pathogens are microorganisms that may produce certain medical conditions, such as chickenpox, measles, mumps, smallpox, or worse, Ebola.

Stress. When you're stressed, you often experience unusual situations, such as having splotchy skin, feeling depressed, having the worst headaches, and extreme mood swings, which you may think are normal but may mean that certain parts of your body are already in too much pain.

3. Chemical, which are often brought forth by stressors that aren't natural to the body, such as:

Alcohol. Some people's lungs and bodies swell when they drink alcohol.

Irritants. Every person reacts different to irritants that may penetrate their body. Irritants are also called allergens—it could range from pollens, pet fur, legumes, dust mites, spores, or basically anything that makes a person itch, have splotches on the body, and have hard time breathing. You can always ask your doctor for an allergen test so you could determine which allergens you should be aware of.

Toxins. Unfortunately, there are a lot of toxins in the food that one eats and the many drinks around—so you really have to be vigilant and whenever you feel irritated or do not feel normal upon eating or drinking something, feel free to see a doctor already.

Other Factors

Moreover, certain conditions such as having elevated C Proteins, High SED Rate, High Homocystine Levels, Elevated Blood Pressure, and an inhibition of Monocytes could also trigger inflammation rate. It could also be brought upon by:

Age. Age is also a factor. More often than not, people who are in their 30's to 50's and older are more susceptible to this condition, because naturally, younger ones have healthier bodies and tougher immune systems. But then again, everyone's bodies are different so no matter how young you are, you still should not just dismiss this condition as something you won't experience at all. Mitochondrial dysfunction can happen to anyone.

Diet. Mostly, people who are overweight, suffering from Diabetes, and those who consume too much saturated fat are in danger of this.

Excess of Glucose. Glucose is tricky. When they're properly consumed by the body, they can be converted to energy, and the body can use it as its own fuel. But then, an excess of glucose has adverse effects to the body, which may destroy cells and bring forth chronic inflammation, especially when they're just accumulated in the bloodstream.

Low Sex Hormones. Unusual low levels of sex hormones not only kills one's sex life, it may also be the cause of inflammation, and bone breakage. It may also produce unusual symptoms of unease during menopause, as well.

Obesity. As mentioned, being overweight is a problem. When metabolism is affected, it already means that chronic inflammation is happening because the body can no longer secrete and store a lot of hormones and blood circulation is also affected, and thus, cells secrete more fat, which then leads to swelling of the body.

Sleeping Disorders. Pro-inflammatory muscles are elevated when one doesn't have a normal circadian rhythm, and when he almost always has a hard time going to sleep, which is also the result of the elevation of plasma in the body. It also happens to those who has narcolepsy and sleep apnea, too.

Smoking. Inflammation is produced by the thousands of chemicals contained in

Now, when your body gets affected by these things, you can expect that you'd suffer from certain diseases, such as Kawasaki Disease, heart ailments, stroke, Diabetes, Cancer, Chronic Lower Respiratory Disease, Alzheimer's Disease, Nephritis, and other Autoimmune Diseases.

So, what you have to do then is change your diet and improve your lifestyle—and it all starts with this book!

Click Here to Check out the Rest of "The Anti Inflammatory Diet" On Amazon

Or go to: **http://amzn.to/1Jf8k66**

Preview From Best Selling Author Jessica Virna "The Truth About Carbs"

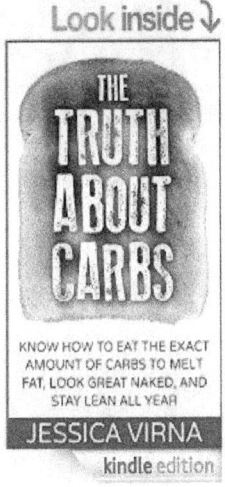

Look inside ↓

THE TRUTH ABOUT CARBS

KNOW HOW TO EAT THE EXACT AMOUNT OF CARBS TO MELT FAT, LOOK GREAT NAKED, AND STAY LEAN ALL YEAR

JESSICA VIRNA

kindle edition

Introduction

I want to thank you and congratulate you for downloading the book, *"The Truth About Carbs: Know How To Eat The Exact Amount Of Carbs To Melt Fat, Look Great Naked, And Stay Lean All Year."*

So many have tried countless dieting regimes — detox, vegan, Paleo, South Beach, etc. — but many had not yet met success in terms of weight loss and achieving a leaner, slimmer figure. What could be the problem? While the ultimate goal is to lose weight, some people have trouble losing *fat*. This book is aimed toward those dieters and anyone who wants to learn how to melt fat and stay lean, by focusing on the ever-elusive, ever-controversial *carbohydrates*.

This book will teach you the *truth* about carbs and how you can deal with this molecule. You don't have to *completely eliminate* carbs and say goodbye to your favorite food groups (never say goodbye to pastries or pasta!). You will learn how to eat carbs the proper way — for the benefit of your health and the success of your fat-loss endeavor.

Click here to check out the Rest of "The Truth About Carbs" on Amazon

Or go to: http://amzn.to/1RFykvc

Preview From Best Selling Author Jessica Virna "Essential Oils Therapy"

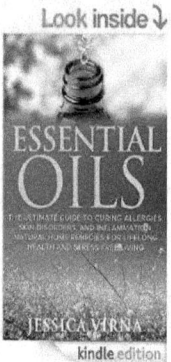

Benefits of Aromatherapy

There are various benefits of aromatherapy and possess different properties. Even if essential oils are good for first aid and relief, they are not enough to take the place of professional medication from licensed healthcare practitioners. Likewise, it is always good measure to have a person checked after providing first aid.

Essential oils can be unassuming but can have many versatile uses in a household. It pays to familiarize yourself with properties of essential oils so that you can act fast and know what needs to be done in case of emergencies.

Benefits

1. Improves skin
2. Helps digestion
3. Promotes sleep and relaxation
4. Natural first aid
5. Aromatherapy

Properties

1. Analgesic-some essential oils can relieve pain such as lavender, black pepper and bergamot.

2. Anesthetic-for emergencies, peppermint, clove, bay and eucalyptus can be used as an anaesthetic.

3. Antimicrobial-anise, bay, cajuput and benzoin along with black pepper have the ability to destroy or suppress microorganism and bacterial growth.

4. Antioxidant-essential oils can help remove damaging oxidizing agents in the body like ginger and benzoin.

5. Antiseptic-there are essential oils that can prevent decay like basil, bay, cedarwood, cinnamon, pine, sage, thyme and ylang ylang.

6. Antispasmodic-clove, cypress, garlic, thyme and basil essential oils can relive the nerves and reduce or prevent excessive muscular spasms and contractions.

7. Carminative-carminative properties mean that an essential oil has the ability to stimulate intestinal peristalsis, and relieve the expulsion of gas from the gastrointestinal tract. Such is the use of cinnamon, coriander, garlic, lemon, black pepper, basil and anise because they tend to introduce *heat* in the body.

8. Disinfectant-there are natural disinfectants in the organic world and the citrus essential oils are always dual purpose, like lemon and orange because of their acidic properties.

9. Stimulant-stimulants increase functional activity and energy in the body, which essential oils like bergamot, juniper, peppermint, jasmine and thyme can do.

10. Tonic- tonics tend to energize and strengthen the body like thyme, yarrow, black pepper, eucalyptus and cajuput.

Essential oils are more than just a good scent and home décor. There are many health benefits that can be derived from these natural wonders. Use your imagination and live a healthier lifestyle, you definitely deserve it.

Click Here to check out the Rest of "Essential Oils Therapy" on Amazon

Or Go to: http://amzn.to/1cUvAdI

Preview From Best Selling Author Jessica Virna "Weight Watchers"

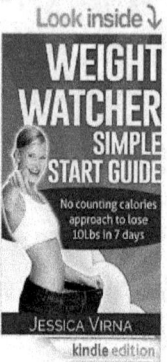

Chapter 1. Weight Watchers and PointsPlus Value

The Weight Watchers® diet program is centered on food that is low in fat but high in fiber. Eat a lot of food within this selection in order to lose 1 to 2 pounds a day. There are times when you may crave for high fat muffins; the Weight Watcher recipes included in this cookbook has low fat and delicious muffins for you to prepare.

This diet program focuses on fruits, vegetables and protein that will enable you to increase your energy. Spend the energy at the gym to gain muscles instead of sitting on a couch the whole day.

Losing 10 lbs. in a week will not be difficult at all! The Weight Watchers® program now boasts of its new and improved PointsPlus values that will guide you to balance your food intake to lose weight. Based on a 1,000 calorie/day diet, you will learn how to eat a filling and balanced meal. Within the PointsPlus directives, you are allowed to consume 26 to 71 points in a day.

Keep in mind that you are not required to eat within the maximum limits that the point guide suggests. This is to give you a non-restrictive diet plan that will not leave you weak while in the process of losing weight.

Physical activity is needed to burn the extra calories that you have gained should you reach the maximum limits of the Weight Watchers® provisionary PointsPlus. In order for you to effectively lose weight, why not try to splurge more on fruits and vegetable? For you see, they have a PointsPlus value of 0. This way, you will feel full without having to think about the calories.

Among the Weight Watchers® dieters, this technique is called the filling technique. They eat designated food that does not add weight and calories. To bring the PointsPlus calorie tracker to a mathematical explanation, you simply would have to allocate points depending on your weight, height, activity level and age.

Aside from the PointsPlus® formula which can be calculated through a link in the website, there is also the ActivityPoints formula wherein you can check as to how many points you can include in your meal plan; based on the level of your physical activities. The more active you are, the higher your PointsPlus allocation is.

Keeping the weight off will not be a problem at all through the help of the Weight Watchers PointsPlus technique. This cookbook will show you the healthy way that the author chose to follow in order to lose 140 lbs.

Click Here to check out the Rest of "Weight Watchers Guide"

Or go to: **http://amzn.to/1G75fnI**

Preview From Best Selling Author Jessica Virna "Buddhism"

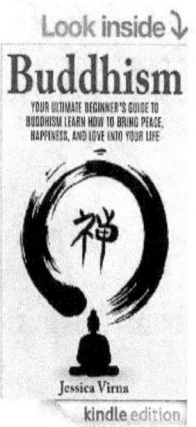

The First Noble Truth: Suffering

The enlightened Buddha realized that life is full of suffering. Whether one looks at his own life or at the world around him, this state is inescapable. The Buddha saw the world of suffering the moment he left the palace. In fact, the pre-conditions to fulfill the prophecy all pointed to different forms of suffering. Through the old man, he saw that everyone would eventually suffer of old age. One's former complexion may fade and wrinkles would surface. His strength would diminish; his capabilities would lessen.

The image of the sick man also portrayed the reality of people being prone to illnesses and diseases. Despite the joys of being healthy, this state wouldn't always be present. One's eyes may begin having difficulty seeing and other body parts may experience pain that wasn't formerly present. Moreover, death could strike anyone at any minute. In seeing the image of the funeral, Siddhartha saw that everyone would experience death.

For someone who was never exposed to pain, all these realities can be very overwhelming. From the moment a child is born until his death, pain would be present. However, these didn't cause Siddhartha to lock himself up in the palace. In fact, the words of the hermit even inspired him to discover more about suffering in the hopes of learning how to achieve happiness.

The first noble truth embraces the inevitability of suffering. Despite the joys and pleasures of life, pain would always appear. However, despite the negativity that this may indicate, the Buddha explains that these are normal. These should not be feared or hated. Rather, people must accept suffering and prepare for it.

Knowing Suffering

Suffering can come in two main forms. First, there is physical pain. This can be seen through harm inflicted on the body. Wounds, fractured legs, or even sickness are indicators of physical harm. Such suffering can be of varying degrees. They can last for as little as a few seconds to even an entire lifetime. However, while most people view suffering to be applicable only to the physical body, the Buddha clarified that this can also emerge in the spirit.

People experience various emotions. These include hate, anger, and greed. People can even feel depressed or lonely. Many of these are unhealthy and unwanted feelings that can affect one's health and disposition. The death of loved ones and other unfortunate events can also trigger such hardships and emotions. Failures and losses can also result to this painful sensation. While these emotions seem to be hidden and minor, they can cause worse effects than physical pain. In fact, they can even elevate the suffering caused by the physical body.

Although people want to experience as little pain as possible, it is clear that this would exist in everyday situations. Even the most minor nuances can trigger suffering. However, the Buddha teaches his followers that these are all natural. Instead of fearing or running away from such emotions, one should slowly and carefully learn to accept these. In fact, knowing suffering would be the key to eventually know happiness.

Of Suffering and Happiness

Although suffering is dominant in life, the Buddha also claims that joy and happiness can also be found simultaneously. Amidst the pain, there can be happiness in friendship, family, health, and other positive factors. These would depend on the perception of an individual. While there are times for suffering, there would also be times of happiness. Buddhists would claim that while both are part of life, these aren't necessarily present permanently. There is some form of balance which can be handled by individuals.

Knowing that suffering and happiness can coexist, the Buddhists proceed to explain that many people make the mistake of trying to escape suffering. They try to distract themselves by indulging in temporary pleasure. Drinking, gambling, and other habits are methods to forget about these unwanted feelings. In their attempt to block out sadness, loss, and grief, they try to delude themselves with pleasure. However, in reality, these wouldn't be effective and would just end up bringing more severe forms of pain and sadness. This would produce worse effects once the temporary happiness perishes. For example, if a person with a cold tries to cheer himself up by eating ice cream, this may just temporarily satisfy his taste buds. After a while, this would contribute to the worsening condition of his colds.

Applying the First Noble Truth

It is important to accept the first truth if one desires to be a step closer to knowing how to gain happiness and enlightenment. Although this teaching may be ancient, this is very applicable to this day and age.

1) **It's okay to be worried, but don't let it control your life.**
   People may get the misconception that the first truth encourages them to stop worrying about bills, insurance, and other things. However, this is incorrect. Fear caused by possible suffering is normal. After all, it's an undesirable state to be in. One shouldn't become boastful and feel invincible to suffering. However, at the same time, one shouldn't let the emotions inflicted by suffering take control of his life. Instead of letting it dictate one's disposition, it should help strengthen one's morale and character. Yes, suffering can sometimes feel too unbearable. However, suffering will always be merely a state that can be overcome. Hence, there is a need to control one's emotions. In effect, he can live life more fully and strive to find happiness.

2) **Prepare for suffering. It will always be there.**
   One shouldn't just offer himself to suffering. Of course, he should find ways to prepare for it or even prevent it from worsening. An individual can choose to plan ahead, ask help from friends, or other methods to cater to his needs. He doesn't have to face suffering unarmed.

3) **Be optimistic.**

   Many people who experience suffering feel as if it indicates the end of the world. They may lose the will to work or even live. These thoughts won't be beneficial in one's pursuit of happiness. Suffering is perfectly normal. Though suffering may hinder a person to fulfill his goals or plans, this doesn't mean that suffering should take control of the rest of his life. One should still think positive amidst the pain he endures. This perhaps is the most effective way to combat such feelings.

4) **Be realistic.**
   Suffering is very real and shouldn't be taken for granted. Hence, one should understand how it can affect his life. Knowing the implications of a certain form of suffering can be helpful as one responds to it. Understanding a certain health illness or consequences of not paying bills can all help the person experiencing problems.

For the Buddha, there is a need to focus on the realities of life. To achieve happiness, one must embrace whatever is happening in life. Distractions would be of temporary benefit but would be inevitably futile. Hence, as both happiness and suffering are both temporary, people must learn to live with these. This is the first step to achieving inner peace and enlightenment. Of course, it doesn't end there. The Buddha then proceeds to discuss the succeeding truths.

Click **Here** to check out the Rest of "BUDDHISM: Your Ultimate Beginner's Guide to Bring Peace, Happiness, and Enlightenment Into Your Daily Life" on Amazon

Or Go To: http://amzn.to/1QK7j8r